I0413453

The Real Cause and Solution for Alcohol Addiction

The NEW Alcoholism Story

Suka Chapel-Horst, RN, Ph.D.

The Real Cause and Solution for Alcohol Addiction
The NEW Alcoholism Story

Author: Suka Chapel-Horst, RN, Ph.D., QMHP, CPLT

Published by:
Brainworks Publishing
638 Spartanburg Highway, Suite #70-175
Hendersonville, NC 28792

www.AriseAlcoholRecovery.com
www.IMRIWellness.org

Neither the publisher nor the author is engaged in rendering professional advice or services to the individual reader. The ideas, procedures, and suggestions contained in this book are not intended as a substitute for consulting with your health care provider. All matters regarding your health require medical supervision. Neither the author nor the publisher shall be liable or responsible for any loss or damage allegedly arising from any information or suggestions in this book.

While the author has made every effort to provide accurate telephone numbers and Internet addresses at the time of publication, neither the publisher nor the author assumes any responsibility for errors, or for changes that occur after publication. Further, the publisher does not have any control over and does not assume any responsibility for author or third-party websites or their content.

ISBN: 10-1494729822
ISBN: 13- 978-1494729820

Copyright © 2013 Suka Chapel-Horst
Copyright © 2015 Suka Chapel-Horst, Revised Edition
Copyright © 2016 Suka Chapel-Horst, Revised Edition

Permission granted to copy or reproduce any portion of this book.

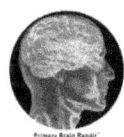 PRIMARY BRAIN REPAIR

Primary Brain Repair focuses on providing the brain, body, and spirit with the basic requirements for health and wellbeing. It's the first line response to all illnesses and disorders. It involves the use of natural micronutrients, nutrition therapy, exercise, and stress relief.

Optimal health can be achieved by most people by following these simple guidelines and these basic health steps will be the foundation for more intensive treatment, if needed.

At Brainworks Recovery, our mission and passion is to educate the public and healthcare professionals about the most advanced methods for obtaining optimal health, naturally. Based on the latest neuroscience and biochemical research, along with years of experience, Dr. Suka offers leading-edge knowledge and how-to information to those who are seeking real recovery versus symptom relief.

Using simple, but effective, recovery tools, *Primary Brain Repair* will improve the health of everyone who applies it. How can that be? Simply, because we go back to the basics of how the brain and body are designed to work. The answer is in nature, and the method is natural.

At Brainworks Recovery we are passionate about helping you. That's why we've created self-help workbooks and DVDs to guide you through the process.

Brainworks Recovery is a non-profit organization.
Our mission is wellness education.

Books and DVDs by Suka Chapel-Horst

WORKBOOKS
How to Quit Drinking for Good and Feel Good

Why Do I Feel This Way?" Natural Healing for Optimal Health and
Relief from Moods and Depression

BOOKS
Take a Leap of Faith

DVD PowerPoint Presentation
Depression Cure – Ten Different Sources / Ten Different Approaches
Your Guide to Finding and Treating the Real Underlying Cause

BOTTOM LINE BOOKS
BOOKS/DVD PowerPoint Presentations
Wellness Simplified – How Food affects Moods, Bodies, and Behaviors

Say Goodbye to Moods and Depression

PTSD – Posttraumatic Stress Disorder, Alternative Resources for Recovery

The Gift – A Sound Mind for Life

Trick or Treat – What Your Doctor isn't Telling You about
Mood Altering Medications

Cannabinoids: Marijuana – The Hundredth Monkey Cure

These books and DVD's can be ordered through:
www.AriseAlcoholRecovery.com
3

ABOUT THE AUTHOR

Dr. Suka has over forty-five years of experience as a Registered Nurse in the fields of mental health, criminal justice, addictions, and wellness education. She worked in hospitals, addiction and detox centers, residential treatment centers for the mentally ill, residential homes for the mentally challenged, locked facilities and residential treatment homes for teenagers with criminal histories. Dr. Suka has been a jail nurse, home health nurse, operating room nurse, infertility education nurse, and owner of a nursing services business serving residential treatment centers.

In 1984 Dr. Suka completed a seminary program and was ordained as an inter-faith minister. This led to training as a hospital chaplain, and to becoming chaplain to a county sheriff's department. Her doctorate is in the ministry.

Dr. Suka is the founder and director of *ARISE* Alcohol Recovery, LLC, offering an out-patient program and two self-help alcohol recovery programs that can be done in the privacy and comfort of one's home while continuing with normal daily activities or work responsibilities.

She is a wellness consultant and a Certified Integrative Memory Therapist, author, and speaker.

INTRODUCTION

Alcohol addiction is a body/mind disorder. Nothing new about that, however our understanding about how brain and body systems work has increased and new forms of talk therapy have evolved since 1935 when Alcoholics Anonymous was the only group addressing the addiction.

Traditional thinking about alcohol addiction is now obsolete. Neuroscience and biochemistry, plus over fifty-five years of experience, have given us a new and far more successful approach to recovery from this debilitating disorder.

The underlying *physical* cause of all addictions is either inherited or acquired imbalanced brain chemistry, and the underlying *mental* cause of all addictions is unconscious, unresolved memories of traumatic experiences. Alcohol does not cause alcohol addiction. When the focus of addiction treatment is on the rebalancing of brain chemistry, plus belief management and memory therapy, recovery rates can soar.

This book explores the most advanced treatment method for recovery now available. While there is always new research and scientific studies on the horizon, we are confident in saying that the information you are about to read is the most advanced recovery system available at this time and we encourage individuals with an addiction to alcohol to seek out programs and practitioners who can provide these advanced treatment methods.

I make no promises of recovery from using this method. Rather, recovery depends upon how committed and dedicated the person with an alcohol addiction is to applying the techniques and strategies offered.

"Dr. Suka" Chapel-Horst, RN, Ph.D.
December 2013
Etowah, North Carolina

CONTENTS

1 ALCOHOL ADDICTION

Recovery without relapse is possible with information, effort and determination.

Let's begin by looking at some facts. Our latest statistics from 2010 show that an estimated 22.1 million people were dependent upon, or were abusing, alcohol and drugs. That's 8.7 percent of the population aged 12 or older.

4.2 million people were using illicit drugs but not alcohol. 2.9 million people were using both alcohol and illicit drugs. 15 million were using alcohol but not illicit drugs. That means that a total of 17.9 million people, or 82%, were abusing or dependent upon alcohol. (*Diagnostic and Statistical Manual of Mental Disorders*, 4th edition [DSM-IV])

Of those 22.1 million people who needed treatment, only 2.6 (<12%) million actually received treatment, leaving 20.5 million who continued to be dependent upon alcohol and drugs, both prescription and illegal drugs.

Traditional recovery methods include 12 Steps, support groups, talk therapy, counseling, and medications. How well is it working?

Up to 95% relapse in the first six to twelve months of sobriety. What are we missing?

Alcohol does not cause alcohol addiction. Bold statement and true. The real underlying causes are three.

THREE UNDERLYING CAUSES OF ALCOHOL ADDICTION

1. Genetically inherited biochemical deficiencies.

2. Environmentally induced biochemical deficiencies, caused, in part, by poverty, malnutrition, toxins, chronic stress, and chronic *abuse* of alcohol.

3. Conscious and unconscious, *unresolved* memories, or stories, of traumatic events.

In the following chapters you'll learn about five biochemical factors affecting an addiction to alcohol (and other drugs, including addictive medications). In a later chapter you will learn about the effects of posttraumatic stress, something we all experience in varying degrees.

2 BIOCHEMICAL FACTOR ONE
Neurotransmitter Imbalances

1) Neurotransmitter Imbalances

Bill Wilson, the co-founder of Alcoholics Anonymous said, "There is a biochemical connection with alcoholism." He was ignored. He was actually told that he would be removed from the board of AA if he continued to attempt to spread that information to the AA community. However, Wilson was correct because alcohol does not cause alcohol addiction.

In 1988 Kenneth Blum, Ph.D., a neuroscientist, along with other scientists, discovered the genetic coding that is the underlying cause of all addictions. He called it a "Reward Deficiency Syndrome". Addictions are the result of a dysfunction in brain chemistry that is completely out of conscious control.

The new addiction story is that addiction is a disease of "brain function." It's not a mental illness. (American Society of Addiction Management [ASAM] 2011)

REWARD DEFICIENCY
The following disorders are partially due to a biochemical imbalance of brain chemistry. (American Society Addiction Medicine 2011)
- Addictions
- ADD/ADHD
- Moods
- Depression
- Tourette's syndrome
- Personality disorders
- Mental disorders
- PTSD

Reward deficiency is also one of the causes of posttraumatic stress disorder (PTSD), for which alcohol, and other drugs, are often used for symptom relief. The recovery model in this book also applies to recovery from PTSD, even if alcohol is not being used for symptom relief.

The biggest cause, and source, of PTSD is UNCONSCIOUS, unresolved trauma which occurred *prior* to the events of the present, known, traumatic experience. (See Chapter 11.)

A reward deficiency can be a primary or an acquired disorder. When the reward deficiency is a *primary* disorder it's due to an inherited genetic dysfunction. Genes are inherited chemical programs that come, half from the father and half from the mother. These programs are encoded in our DNA and they are protein recipes for our neurotransmitter levels.

When the reward deficiency is an *acquired* disorder, the brain chemistry dysfunction can be due to:
- Allergies
- Toxic metals
- Candida yeast
- MALNUTRITION (huge issue in the U.S.)
- Molds / Chemicals both ingested and inhaled
- Gut impermeability letting poisons in and keeping nutrients out
- Hormone imbalances
- Alcohol / Drug ABUSE
- CHRONIC STRESS

BRAIN CHEMISTRY

There are about 100 billion neurons in the brain but they're not physically connected to each other. Communication occurs through chemicals that carry messages from one neuron to another. These chemicals are called neurotransmitters and there are over a 100 of them. Neurotransmitters are made of food proteins and proteins are made up of amino acids, a point to remember.

There are four main neurotransmitters that affect addictions.

Dopamine is the "Energizer Bunny" neurotransmitter. It's a "feel good" chemical. It stimulates and excites us.

Serotonin is the "Happy Sunshine" neurotransmitter. It's a relaxer. It's responsible for our moods, our sleep, appetite, and perception.

GABA is the "Chill Out" neurotransmitter. It's a sedative and it reduces anxiety.

Endorphins are the "Love Bug" neurotransmitters. They bring us comfort and pleasure. They are the brain's natural pain killers, for both emotional and mental pain.

Dopamine Deficiency ("Feel good" chemical that stimulates and excites) Energizer Bunny Neurotransmitter

Symptoms of a Dopamine deficiency are:
- Reduced ability to feel pleasure
- Flat, bored, apathetic and low enthusiasm
- Depressed
- Low drive and motivation
- Procrastination
- Difficulty concentrating
- Slowed thinking
- Low energy
- Shyness/introversion
- Low libido or impotence
- Sleep too much
- Restless leg syndrome
- Trouble getting out of bed
- Put on weight easily
- Easily mentally and physically fatigued
- Family history of alcoholism/AD(H)D

Typical Dopamine Deficiency Solutions that are used to get the missing reward.

- Cocaine
- Crack
- Amphetamines
- Methamphetamine
- Marijuana
- Adderall Ritalin Concerta
- Caffeine
- Tobacco
- ALCOHOL

Serotonin Deficiency (Emotional Relaxer affecting moods, sleep, appetite, and perception) "Happy Sunshine" Neurotransmitter

Symptoms of a Serotonin deficiency are:
- Depression
- Irritability
- Impatience
- Impulsiveness
- Inability to concentrate
- Weight gain or unexplained weight loss
- Slow growth in children
- Poor dream recall
- Insomnia

Typical Serotonin Deficiency Solutions that are used to get the missing reward.

- Marijuana
- Antidepressants
- Sleep aids
- Tobacco
- ALCOHOL

GABA Deficiency (Mental relaxation, sedative, reduces anxiety, feel good) "Chill Out" Neurotransmitter

Symptoms of a GABA deficiency are:
- Anxiety, difficulty relaxing
- Easily stressed or overwhelmed
- Overworked or pressured
- Body uptight or stiff
- Sometimes feel weak or shaky
- Increased stress if skip a meal
- Bothered by loud noises, lights, too much activity

Typical GABA Deficiency Solutions that are used to get the missing reward.
- Benzodiazepines (Sedative hypnotics - Valium, Ativan, Xanax, Klonipin, Restoril, etc.)
- Barbiturates (Fioricet for migraines)
- Sleep Aids (Ambien, Lunesta, Prosom)
- Tobacco
- Marijuana
- ALCOHOL

Endorphin Deficiency (Natural pain killers, comfort, pleasure) "Love Bug" Neurotransmitter

Actually, the endorphins are a group of chemicals that act *like* neurotransmitters. Symptoms of an endorphin deficiency are:
- Discomfort
- Persistent emotional pain
- Persistent physical pain
- Over sensitivity
- Stress and frustration

Typical Endorphin Deficiency Solutions that are used to get the missing reward.

- OPIATES (Heroin, Percocet, OxyContin, Hydrocodone)
- Methadone (synthetic opiate)
- Suboxone (synthetic opiate)
- Marijuana
- Tobacco
- ALCOHOL

People with a reward deficiency don't experience the same *internal* rewards, or good feelings, that people with normal brain chemistry do. They're *"reward deficient"*.

There is no such a thing as a "drug of choice." People don't "choose" their drug because drugs mimic natural brain chemistry. People will use, and abuse, the drug that provides the missing reward.

However, alcohol dependent people are deficient in ALL FOUR neurotransmitters. That's why the majority of addicted people use alcohol to self-medicate.

Corticotrophin-Releasing Hormone (CRH) is a hormone that acts **like** a neurotransmitter. It manages the body's response to stress and anxiety. People who are predisposed to an alcohol addiction don't handle stress well because they have inherited a CRH deficiency. CRH, as well, is due to an inherited, genetic, protein recipe resulting in an amino acid deficiency.

Almost all alcohol addicted people will tell you that they always felt different from other people while they were growing up.

Addictions are unconscious physiological attempts to create the "feel good" reward that is naturally missing from the brain. As the addiction progresses, it becomes an unconscious physiological REQUIREMENT for survival, overriding all conscious attempts to stop the addiction.

Addiction is NOT about will power. It is NOT about shame. It is NOT about guilt. It IS about PHYSICAL SURVIVAL. It is BEYOND the mind and conscious control.

Alcohol ABUSERS WANT to drink. They can stop drinking if they WANT to stop. Alcohol ADDICTED people HAVE to drink to survive. They CAN'T stop.

REWARD PATHWAY

The front and outermost part of the brain is called the neocortex. It's where we think, using words and numbers. This part of the brain can intuit, analyze, foresee the consequences of actions, discriminate, and can choose to be socially responsible.

The limbic system lies in the center of the brain. It's also called the mammalian brain because it's in all mammals. It's a primitive brain that doesn't have words or language. It responds only to the five senses: sight, sound, feeling, hearing, and taste and this is where memories and all emotions reside and it's where the reward pathway is found.

The limbic system is a primitive brain that has only one purpose, and that is to survive. It's all about fight or flight responses. Let me give you an example.

We know that if we don't have enough oxygen, we will die in just a few minutes. So why is it that when the lungs of drowning victims are examined, there is always water in the lungs? A drowning person knows he will die if he gets water in his lungs, so why would he breathe? No matter how hard he tries not to breathe, the limbic system will cause him to open his mouth and breathe. He will suck in water and die.

The limbic system doesn't know about water. It only knows that it has to breathe in oxygen or it will die and so it breathes. It does what it has to do to survive, unaware that it will cause death in this instance. This is the survival response of a primitive brain.

So let's look at the reward pathway, located in this primitive brain. Laura drinks alcohol to get a reward. Perhaps she has felt depressed all during her childhood. She's found that alcohol makes her feel more normal, happier, and more outgoing.

As she drinks, the alcohol raises her dopamine level. That's why she feels so good. Dopamine is the "feel good" neurotransmitter. But, with prolonged, frequent drinking, too much dopamine can be released into the brain and the brain experiences a dopamine overload. This can cause hyperthermia, raising the temperature from 103 to 107 degrees and this would cause her death.

So Laura's brain, always survival oriented, decreases the amount of dopamine it produces in order to maintain a balance, even though her level of dopamine was lower than normal to begin with. Also, receptors on the receiving neurons begin to close down, to avoid an overload. Now, it takes even more alcohol to stimulate a dopamine release.

This means that Laura no longer gets the reward of feeling good. She's back to feeling like she did before she started drinking. We call that "tolerance." But the kicker is that now she can't stop drinking because she needs the alcohol to stimulate a dopamine release in order to function at all. Her brain has become dependent upon the alcohol. Her brain is producing less and less dopamine the longer she drinks. Laura now NEEDS the alcohol to stimulate a dopamine release in order to just survive.

The brain, now producing very small amounts of dopamine feels like it is dying. Laura will feel desperation and gut wrenching cravings which her mind can't control. It has become a life or death situation. The alcohol Laura needs in order to survive is killing her.

Will power cannot override survival needs. The primitive brain is in control craving what it needs in order to stimulate the neurotransmitters that are needed for survival. It's a "catch 22".

Blame, guilt, and shame are out of place. Compassion for Laura's struggle to survive is the only legitimate reaction.

Sobriety is not recovery. One day at a time is not recovery. White-knuckling is not recovery. Mood swings are not recovery.

WHY CAN'T THEY JUST STOP DRINKING?

So, how is it that some people can just quit drinking and others relapse over and over? The answer lies in the DEGREE of reward deficiency a person has.

Cheryl may have a severe deficiency in her neurotransmitters and is dependent upon alcohol to stimulate enough dopamine just to survive. If she stops drinking, cold turkey, her brain will force her to crave the alcohol in order to get enough dopamine, for example, just to continue to survive. She is on automatic pilot. No matter what, without proper treatment, she needs alcohol just to stay alive. It truly is life or death.

That's why people will do anything to get their alcohol and that's why we should not judge them poorly. They are trying to survive and it's all a function of the primitive, but necessary part of the brain, NOT the mind. It truly is life or death.

On the other hand, Matt, who is a long time drinker with all the symptoms of addiction, can quit, if he determines to do so. Matt has been abusing alcohol for years but, fortunately for him, his neurotransmitter levels are not so severely deficient. His brain is still producing enough dopamine, for example, to keep him going. He is not in survival mode, even though he craves the alcohol and feels sick when he doesn't have it.

Nevertheless, Matt has been drinking long enough that he exhibits all the emotional reactions and behaviors of a serious addiction. However, when he finally decides to quit drinking, his conscious mind, his neocortex, is still able to override his primitive brain's impulses. How fortunate for him.

Matt stops drinking and, hopefully, also addresses the results of his long years of drinking. What's important here is that just because he was able to quit drinking doesn't mean everyone else can. The statement some recovering people make is "If I did it, you can too." Not so. It all depends upon the level of brain chemical deficiencies a person was born with. In other words, what is the degree of reward deficiency?

This explains the relapse rate people experience, regardless of where they seek help. If the support group or treatment facility is not addressing biochemical deficiencies, those people with more severe deficiencies will relapse unless they get the proper treatment.

What is the proper treatment? Read on.

3 AMINO ACID THERAPY

Talk and talk therapy do NOT restore neurotransmitter levels. Relapse is a survival mechanism of the old brain.

The good news is that recovery without relapse is possible when biochemical imbalances are treated. The recovery solution is to restore neurotransmitters, hormones, and gut permeability to normal. (95% of Serotonin is made in the gut.) A healthy gut is necessary for proper absorption of nutrients from supplements and food.

Neurotransmitter recovery begins with amino acids. Amino acids are proteins and neurotransmitters are made from amino acids, not medications! It's an all-natural recovery process.

NEUROTRANSMITTER REPLACEMENT
Relapse-free recovery requires neurotransmitter recovery so here's a reminder about those four major neurotransmitters.

Dopamine and **serotonin** *feel* like *"uppers."* They lift us up and make us feel better. Dopamine energizes, excites, and can make us feel euphoric. Serotonin feels like sunshine, making us happier and more flexible.

GABA and the **endorphins** *feel* like *"downers.* GABA decreases anxiety, and helps us to chill out. The endorphins decrease physical and emotional pain by decreasing anger, sensitivity, unhappiness, and loneliness.

ALCOHOL

- Alcohol **energizes** us by stimulating the release of Dopamine.

- Alcohol makes us **happy** by stimulating the release of Serotonin.

- Alcohol **relaxes** us by stimulating the release of GABA.

- Alcohol reduces **pain** by stimulating the release of the Endorphins.

AMINO ACIDS

So, let's switch the alcohol addiction to an amino acid addiction. Here's why.

- The amino acid, L-Tyrosine, **rebuilds** low dopamine levels.

- The amino acid, L- Tryptophan, **rebuilds** low serotonin levels.

- The amino acid, GABA, **rebuilds** low GABA levels.

- The amino acid, DL-Phenylalanine, **rebuilds** low endorphins levels, (plus other amino acids and co-factors)

ADVANTAGES OF AMINO ACID THERAPY

- Cravings gone

- Anxiety gone

- Depression gone

- Insomnia gone .... all within days!!!

It takes approximately twelve to twenty-four months to rebuild neurotransmitters, depending on the degree of deficiency. 95% of relapse is due to failure to rebuild neurotransmitters. Alcohol addiction is a deadly disorder. It takes time and effort. Don't expect a cure in 90 days.

The workbook, *How to Quit Drinking for Good and Feel Good,* has all the guidelines for neurotransmitter testing, amino acid precautions, and formulas for recovery.

4 BIOCHEMICAL FACTOR TWO - Hypoglycemia

1) Neurotransmitter Imbalances
2) Hypoglycemia

100% of alcoholics are hypoglycemic meaning that they have low blood sugar. Insulin is released in order to metabolize the alcohol and other sugars a person is eating. When a lot of alcohol, or sugar, is being consumed on a regular basis, there is an overproduction of insulin which cries out for more sugar. When a person has low blood sugar they experience:

- Cravings
- Depression
- Unprovoked anxieties
- Exhaustion
- Mental confusion
- Forgetfulness
- Irritability
- Insomnia
- Constant worrying
- Internal trembling

When Scott has normal glucose, or blood sugar levels, flooding his entire brain, he will have the mental ability to be socially responsible. But if he has low blood sugar, the glucose will go to the part of the brain that keeps him alive. He will then be in survival mode with fight or flight, gut reactions. These can include anger and violence, even manslaughter and suicide.

Road rage, domestic violence, and unintended suicide are examples of the actions of people who are in a severe hypoglycemic state, which explains the suicides of many high-functioning teenagers. Too much sugar, sodas, junk and fast foods.

Hypoglycemic symptoms are identical to what's called the dry drunk syndrome (now called "Chronic Abstinence Symptoms"). The suddenly sober addict will stuff himself with coffee, sugar, pizza, pasta, doughnuts, and all forms of sweets to replace the missing alcohol. (Caffeine stimulates the release of emergency sugar which requires the replacing of it by the consumption of more sugar.) Some experts say that the biggest reason for relapse is failure to treat and inform the addict about hypoglycemia.

Sugar is in all the white foods such as:
- Ice cream
- Pasta
- White bread
- Pizza crust
- White rice
- White potatoes
- White flour baked goods

Cross addictions are common. For example: people will switch their alcohol addiction to sugar, nicotine, marijuana or other drugs. If optimum neurotransmitter and biochemical levels are not restored, the primitive brain remains in survival mode. The result: cravings, switching of addictions, dry-drunk behaviors, and *RELAPSE*.

5 FIRST STEPS TO RECOVERY

The first step to recovery should be testing. The book *How to Quit Drinking for Good and Feel Good* by Dr. Suka Chapel-Horst (see Appendix) includes ten written tests to determine any underlying issues that have to be addressed for a relapse-free recovery. These tests include:

- Alcohol screening
- Carbohydrate addiction
- Hypoglycemia
- Candida
- Allergies
- Hypothyroid
- Pyroluria
- High histamine
- Low histamine
- ADD / ADHD
- Adrenal insufficiency

Some suggested laboratory testing: (See Appendix for testing laboratories.)

- CBC Complete Blood Count
- CMP Comprehensive Metabolic Panel
- A1c Testing for diabetes and prediabetes
- Urinalysis
- Thyroid: TSH, Free T3, FreeT4
- 24 hour glucose tolerance test
- Neurotransmitter levels
- DHEA level
- Vitamin D level
- Hormone levels, especially in women
- Copper/Zinc levels
- Toxic metals – Hair or blood analysis

The underlying problem for endorphin-deficient people is that many have very real pain that needs to be addressed in addition to the addiction issue. Unfortunately, many of the alternative methods for pain management are not covered by insurance plans, nor are they even suggested by many physicians.

In addition to treating the alcohol addiction, any co-existing diagnosis must be addressed, including medical complications and a pre-existing mental diagnosis.

Is the solution medications? Medications can provide fast symptom relief but the symptom relief is short term. Side effects require more medications. All mood altering medications are addictive and do not restore brain chemistry. In fact, they further distort brain chemistry.

(In the Appendix see the Book/DVD *Trick or Treat* for information about what your doctor isn't telling you about mood-altering medications.)

6 BIOCHEMICAL FACTOR THREE
Co-Factor Deficiencies

1) **Neurotransmitter Imbalances**
2) **Hypoglycemia**
3) **Co-factor Deficiencies**

Co-factors, or **micronutrients** include:
- Vitamins
- Minerals
- Essential fatty acids
- Enzymes
- Trace elements

How important are these micronutrients? Let's just look at the effects of a vitamin B deficiency.

Emotional Symptoms of a Vitamin B Deficiency
- Mood swings
- Confusion
- Poor memory
- Depression
- Insomnia
- Anxiety
- Obsessive-compulsive behaviors
- Impulsive
- Poor concentration
- Anger
- Irritability
- Quarrelsome
- Panic attacks

Physical Symptoms of a Vitamin B Deficiency

- Hyperactivity
- Headache
- Fatigue
- Insomnia
- Convulsions
- Agitation
- Decreased sex drive
- Tension
- Dizziness
- Gastric ulcers
- High blood pressure
- High cholesterol
- Arteriosclerosis
- Constipation
- Hair loss
- Skin eruptions
- Kidney /Liver impairment
- Extreme nervous exhaustion

Amino acids need vitamin B's to metabolize and rebuild neurotransmitters. Note that alcohol flushes amino acids and vitamin B's out of the body, so it should be no surprise that the addicted person has lots of symptoms.

7 BIOCHEMICAL FACTOR FOUR - Malnutrition

1) **Neurotransmitter Deficiencies**
2) **Hypoglycemia**
3) **Co-factor Deficiencies**
4) **Malnutrition**

People with an alcohol addiction are malnourished. Alcohol makes them feel full so they aren't hungry and they don't eat well. They usually have an inability to metabolize food due to intestinal imbalances. Alcohol also flushes out the some of the nutrients. Many addicted people are living on junk food and fast food. (They're the same, aren't they?)

It's important to **eat three wholesome meals every day**. That means three, not two, or one. The most important meal is breakfast. Studies show that missing breakfast is a sure path to relapse.

After several hours of sleep and no food, Michele will be hypoglycemic in the morning. If she doesn't eat breakfast, she will start craving sweets and be drawn to alcohol to meet the sugar cravings. It's all downhill from there.

Eat lots of protein, healthy fats, fruits, vegetables, some grains, and nuts.

It's very important to **address allergies**. People who binge-drink often have allergies to the grains used to make the alcohol. Wheat and dairy are the most common allergies. If allergies aren't addressed, relapse is almost assured. Are you beginning to understand why just getting sober rarely works?

Eight Most Common Food Allergens

- Wheat

- Milk

- Eggs

- Soy

- Fish

- Shell fish

- Peanuts

- Tree nuts

It's important to **treat hypoglycemia and candida**, a yeast overgrowth in the intestine that is common to alcohol addicted people. Both can cause such an intense craving for sugar that relapse is swift and powerful.

The workbook *How to Quit Drinking for Good and Feel Good* has guidelines for identifying and treating both allergies and Candida.

Drinking six to eight glasses of water daily is extremely important. The nervous system operates well only when the water table is full. We are about 70% water and a low level of water in the body causes many of the chronic symptoms we experience. Caffeinated beverages flush water from the system so you can't count your coffee, and other caffeinated beverages, as water.

8 BIOCHEMICAL FACTOR FIVE - Tobacco

1) Neurotransmitter Deficiencies
2) Hypoglycemia
3) Co-factor Deficiencies
4) Malnutrition
5) Tobacco

The fifth biochemical hindrance to recovery is tobacco. Tobacco is an energizer because it stimulates dopamine. But it also depletes serotonin making one feel down, and, it inhibits GABA which causes anxiety.

When I worked in treatment facilities, it was interesting to watch the behavior of patients when they were deprived of their smoking. They would slam doors, use foul language, verbally attack the staff, and even demand to be released from the program. You could see the effects of nicotine deprivation. They were, literally, operating from the survival part of the brain which was screaming for the drug that gave them the emotional reward they were missing.

Tobacco and relapse are twins. Studies show that almost 100% of those who fail to give up their nicotine will relapse. Of course, giving up two substances, alcohol and nicotine, at the same time is hugely difficult. It's better to continue to smoke while the brain is beginning to rebalance with the micro-nutrients and healthy nutrition. A good time to begin the nicotine withdrawal is about four weeks after beginning a recovery program. By that time, the brain and body will be healthier and can handle the biochemical changes better.

When giving up tobacco, there are a number of added supplements and nutritional guidelines that will help ease the transition.

9 MORE OF THE PICTURE

Exercise or walking

Exercise, or walking, is a MUST for relapse-free recovery. It's a major part of keeping the mind and body alive, alert, and healthy. However, I know that many people don't like to exercise. For those who do, fine. For those who don't, thirty minutes a day or forty minutes of brisk walking every other day will do it. Keeping the heart rate up and breaking a little sweat is a good sign that you're getting a decent workout.

Infra-Red Dry-Heat Saunas

As alcohol metabolizes, it releases toxins into the fatty tissues of the body. In addition, toxins have been accumulating in the body over years. If these toxins aren't removed, they can be released under times of stress. As the toxins enter the blood stream and go to the brain, they can trigger the reward pathway.

Old deeply imbedded memories can cause automatic responses in the limbic system to crave alcohol so intensely that a person can find oneself drinking and not know why or how it happened. This can happen even after years of sobriety.

To avoid future relapse due to toxins and alcohol metabolites stored in the fatty tissues, saunas five days a week for several weeks will assist in removing these toxins from the body.

The lower temperatures of the infra-red dry-heat saunas are preferred to steam saunas because many addicted people have high blood pressure. A few minutes of sweating daily, followed by a soap and water shower to remove the toxins from the skin, is usually all that is needed. I recommend taking these saunas for about four weeks before reducing to just a few times a month.

There are also many natural methods for detoxing the body, including herbal remedies.

Some people are allergic to chemicals in soaps and cosmetics, airborne molds, grasses, and pesticides, for example. It may be necessary to get testing for these substances, as well.

Additional Help

All of the following methods are excellent and can be incorporated in a sound recovery program. I recommend a full-body massage twice a week for the first four to six weeks to remove toxins and begin the relaxation process that must take place for energy blockages to be released. Massage also begins the process of connecting with another human being through touch, encouraging the process of "letting go and letting God (or Spirit)".

- Massage
- Biofeedback
- Auricular therapy
- Acupuncture
- Acupressure
- Cranial-Sacral therapy
- Reflexology
- Yoga
- Meditation
- Other...

10 STAGES OF TREATMENT

Alcohol addiction is responsible for multiple emotional, mental, relationship, and work-related problems. While rehabilitation treatment must embrace these issues, there is no point in attempting psychological therapy until the brain is beginning to recover.

Early in treatment recovering people can't focus, concentrate, or remember very well and they are already under a high degree of stress. Some are still smoking or chewing tobacco in the early stages.

While drinking, or perhaps even before the drinking became established, they shut down their emotions and dug deeply into their survival routines and habits. Give them a few weeks to get their "sea legs" going (neurotransmitter rejuvenation and body system repair).

In the early stages, it is useful to focus on the physical aspects of recovery. Mark needs to learn how to maintain his amino acid and co-factor protocol, on his own, independent of nurses or significant others.

He needs to spend time in the grocery store learning how to purchase healthy foods and then, he needs to spend time learning how to fix his own simple and easy, healthy meals; meals that he enjoys eating.

Mark's time should be spent getting his massages, saunas, swimming if he likes, exercising in the gym, walking, practicing yoga, and learning how to meditate. He needs to sleep and learn how to follow normal waking and sleeping hours. TV, newspapers, computers, and telephones should be unavailable during this time.

It goes without saying that Mark can no longer associate with his drinking buddies. He will need to find non-drinking friends and new activities to replace the time he formerly spent with his best friend, the bottle.

During the early days of recovery treatment, Mark's mind needs to be focused on addiction education, including the causes of addiction, the long range results of continued drinking, and the positive results of recovery.

Mark needs positive, encouraging support during this time. Guilt and shame based talk is counterproductive. Remember, Mark isn't to blame for his addiction. If he hadn't been born with brain chemistry imbalances, he would not be addicted (the majority of addiction is due to inherited brain chemical deficiencies.)

In these early days and weeks, Mark needs to be introduced to his own behavioral responses, the beliefs he holds that are holding him back, and affirmative, positive changes he can make to begin the letting go of ingrained survival responses (belief management training).

Once his brain fog has cleared somewhat, and Mark is feeling physically and emotionally better, he is ready to begin therapy. But don't rush it. Some issues will naturally resolve just because his brain and body are getting healthier. Mark is going to begin to feel good in just days if he is following this program.

Talk therapy will be most productive after Mark has had some time to restore his physical brain and body enough that he is able to focus and concentrate; when he is trusting enough to begin to let down his defenses and allow his true emotions to be expressed. Only when he feels cared for, listened to, and respected, will he be willing to move beyond his long-held denials and face his truths.

There are several therapy models that have proved beneficial for recovery. A therapeutic modality I recommend, that goes to the deepest, underlying source responsible for addictions, and PTSD, is called *Integrative Memory Therapy*® (See next chapter.)

11 POST TRAUMATIC STRESS and PTSD
Third Cause of Alcohol Addiction

1) Genetic Neurotransmitter Deficiencies
2) Acquired Neurotransmitter Deficiencies
3) Post Traumatic Stress and PTSD

Present day physical, emotional, and mental pain, and suffering, are the result of unresolved traumatic experiences from our past.   The unresolved trauma might be relatively small and insignificant, with minor ongoing effects or it can be extremely debilitating with long lasting outward effects, or anywhere in between.

Nevertheless, the lack of resolution causes ongoing, or chronic internal stress that affects our reactions and behavior toward ourselves and others. It affects how we respond to situations that trigger the known or often hidden memory. I call it, *posttraumatic* stress, and we all experience it to varying degrees.   The internal, unresolved memories, even if forgotten, affect our brain and body chemistry.   If unconscious, chronic stress continues, without resolution, it eventually leads to unhealthy emotional and mental reactions, and eventually to physical illness and disease.

For example, if we haven't worked through stressful experiences such as being fired, or from causing hurt to another, or feeling betrayed by a trusted friend, or from the loss of a loved one, we are experiencing posttraumatic stress. A mother may grieve over the loss of a child for years without resolving her pain. This can lead to irritability, anger, depression, insomnia, isolation, divorce, gastric and intestinal disorders, or cancer. This is an example of the effects of posttraumatic stress, due to a failure to resolve the hurt and move forward.

Posttraumatic stress *disorder* (PTSD) is a higher degree of reactions due to unresolved, remembered experiences of severe trauma. Reactions include memories and nightmares, flashbacks, avoidance of things related to the event, severe anxiety, sleeplessness, aggressive behavior and angry outbursts which can strike at any time, most commonly when he or she is reminded of the events in question.

The symptoms of unresolved, conscious and unconscious memories of pain and trauma are one of the causes of alcohol addiction. Alcohol abuse and addiction are frequently co-diagnosed with PTSD.

Alcohol, mood and mind altering pharmaceutical medications, and illegal drugs, serve to cover up or alleviate unwanted symptoms and memories, at least temporarily.

Unresolved traumatic events may have occurred weeks, months, or years ago. These unresolved memories also include all that we saw, heard, and felt during the first seven years of our life, and while we were in the womb. Yes, we recorded the feelings, thoughts, and words mother experienced during the time we were a tiny fetus in her womb. We simply recorded these in our unconscious mind.

These experiences, from our mother in the womb, and from the first seven years of our life, became our history and our truths because we didn't yet have a conscious mind to discriminate. The stories dictated beliefs to us about how to live in the world, even though the beliefs may have been wrong or harmful.

Sometimes these memories or "stories" may appear to be past life trauma stories that are seeking resolution. It makes no difference whether the stories are fantasy or real, if they happened to us or to mother, or to someone else. If they are in *our* unconscious mind, they become *our* stories, and we will live out the lessons we learned from those stories, even if the lessons are not in our own best interest as we go through life.

When *traumatic* stories in the conscious and unconscious mind are left unresolved, they create unhealthy survival patterns which lead to suffering in our present day life. Those survival patterns, which initially occurred at the time of the earlier trauma, are repeated in our present life when we have similar experiences. Because we haven't resolved the earlier traumatic experience, we continue to re-enact our responses to it in the present.

Emotionally, these survival patterns can show up as anxiety, worry, depression, withdrawal, avoidance, PTSD, addictions, overworking, over exercising, competitiveness, anger, fighting, or violence, for example.

Mentally, these survival patterns can create a victim mentality blaming others, stubbornness, self-righteousness, or superiority, to give just a few examples.

Physically, survival patterns can be the cause of anorexia, diabetes, frequent accidents, digestive disorders, or cancer, for example. In fact, every illness and every disorder is the result of both conscious and unconscious unresolved prior trauma.

Integrative Memory Therapy® is a methodology that gets to the originating source of present day issues, allowing for healing and transformation. Unlike other medical and alternative modalities, this process resolves the root of the problem, the unconscious memories of trauma that are controlling present day reactions and behaviors. Healing in the present takes place because the underlying cause is no longer driving behaviors.

Integrative Memory Therapy® is not regression, nor is it hypnosis. Clients are fully conscious at all times. The therapist guides clients to completely resolve their own source trauma. The result is a transformed life in the present. (This therapy must be conducted in person. It cannot be conducted via Skype or telephone.)

To read testimonials and learn more about *Integrative Memory Therapy*® go to www.AriseAlcoholRecovery.com or contact Dr. Suka at 417-890-3254.

12 AFTERCARE

POST-ACUTE WITHDRAWAL SYNDROME (PAWS)

PAWS begins about three weeks after becoming sober and is responsible for quick relapse. People experience high amounts of stress due to all the biochemical changes going on in the brain. If you recall, they have a lowered amount of the CRH (Corticotrophin-Releasing Hormone) so they experience increased stress and over-stimulated senses, much more so than most people.

PAWS SYMPTOMS

- Increased stress

- Over-stimulated senses

- Depression

- Mood swings

- Anxiety

- Sudden panic

- Over and under reactions

- Poor concentration

- Poor memories

- Frequent nightmares

- Slow reflexes

- Dizzy, clumsy, unsteady

- CHRONIC STRESS, STRESS, and MORE STRESS

When alcohol quickly relieves these symptoms so well, is it any surprise that people relapse?

The good news is that when recovering individuals follow a healthy program that rebalances brain chemistry with the amino acid micronutrients, co-factors, and healthy nutrition, PAWS is greatly reduced. In fact, cravings can be gone in just days. This removes a major cause for relapse.

Treat the CAUSE, no more PAWS

AD(H)D

It's believed that 50% to 70%, or more, of people with an alcohol addiction have undiagnosed AD(H)D. When they were in their teens, they may have used alcohol to manage the AD(H)D symptoms, not knowing they had the disorder.

When they quit drinking, all those symptoms come roaring back and these individuals think their symptoms are due to withdrawal. AD(H)D can't be cured but it can be controlled, naturally, with the use of amino acids, and the co-factors. Medications make the condition worse over time. If people aren't aware that they may have AD(H)D, they can easily slip back into the comfort of alcohol.

"I'LL JUST HAVE ONE LITTLE DRINK"

"Can I ever drink again?" The answer is a resounding "NO". Here's why. Think back to the limbic system and the walnut sized amygdala in the reward pathway. You'll remember that this little gland automatically responds to the five senses and processes memories. It doesn't think. Let me give you an example of how this works.

Matt, who's in recovery, is walking through the airport and passes by one of the many bars. He **smells** the alcohol in the air, **hears** the clinking of glasses and the laughter and chatter of the patrons, **sees** the alcohol bottles and flickering beer signs, **feels** his heart beating, and gets the familiar **taste** of his favorite drink in his mouth.

Memories of drinking are released into Matt's primitive brain along with the survival message that is replaying, "I need alcohol to stimulate my brain chemistry in order to survive." Before he can even think, he's sitting at the bar with a drink in his hand. He isn't even aware of what's he's doing. But his brain thinks its survival needs are being met. It's a vicious trick of the brain.

Once started, Matt has no control over how much he drinks. Just one drink and he will be drinking even more than he was drinking before he became sober. Matt isn't drinking because he lost his will power, or because he failed to call his sponsor. He's automatically responding to a survival mechanism that requires an immediate reward which is also completely out of his conscious mind. Please have compassion for him.

Once again, this survival mechanism, while very active for the first twelve to twenty-four months, will be greatly subdued by feeding the brain what it needs to recover; the amino acids, co-factors, healthy nutrition, and other tools. I'm repeating this because recovery insists upon sticking with the program. It's a matter of survival.

BIOCHEMICAL REHABILITATION REVIEW
- Micronutrients for 12 to 24 months for complete brain chemistry repair (amino acids and co-factors)
- Maintain healthy nutrition
- Exercise/walking
- Continue healthy lifestyle including getting adequate sleep

It's all too easy to stop taking the amino acid protocol and micronutrients, and to start eating those unhealthy foods once again. So easy to stop exercising and let down one's guard. Easy to visit those old drinking buddies just to catch up on old times. Bingo. Drink in hand. Relapse. Recovery over.

Very early into this program, Cate started to feel so good that she didn't think she needed to continue her recovery plan. She wasn't drinking, had no cravings, wasn't depressed, and was sleeping like a log. Her relationships were improving and she was beginning to feel proud of herself and optimistic about her future. Cate thought she was cured, but she wasn't. She still had a long way to go to rebuild her neurotransmitters and bodily systems.

This is a most precarious time for Cate. If she stops her recovery program, she will soon relapse and get the mistaken belief that the program didn't work. The truth is, Cate would have gone on to full recovery had she continued her recovery program for the 12 to 24 months that are necessary for full recovery.

Don't be fooled by good feelings.
Stick with the recovery program and feel good, for good.

SUPPORT

Support is absolutely necessary. It can come from a recovered friend, a recovery support group, counseling and therapy, and from spiritual sources. However, it's important for the support people to be in harmony with the biochemical approach to recovery.

Anyone who suggests that the individual has made poor choices, and is consciously responsible for the addiction, will not be helpful. After all, if someone tells me I failed because of my lack of will power, and then blames me for relapsing, I just want to drink some more to stifle my emotions. Choose only those people who will support one's biochemical recovery program.

SUMMARY

These, then, are the tools for a relapse-free recovery.

- Amino acids

- Supplements/Co-factors

- Healthy nutrition

- Walking / Exercise

- Saunas

- Massage

- Alternative healing methods

- Stress management (belief management, therapy, counseling)

- Support

Alcohol addiction is a powerful foe but you've just been given powerful tools, all natural, that are more than up to the challenge. The next step is to make a decision. Recovery without relapse is possible when individuals are **determined to do anything to recover**. That's the ultimate key. I wish for you, or your loved one, complete success. Believe.

13 SELECTING A TREATMENT PROGRAM

Some people can follow a program of recovery at home because they are still highly functioning, both mentally and physically, and they are also highly motivated.   (See Appendix for Dr. Suka's Self-Help Recovery Programs.)

Others may benefit from an out-patient program and still others are best served by a residential treatment program in order to get away from their drinking buddies, or from their private drinking space. They may need separation from a high-drama emotional environment, and they may need to be away from temptation by being in an alcohol-free environment.

If a person does need the benefit of a residential program, be sure that it offers a biochemical approach to recovery. If it doesn't, relapse will likely occur within the first six to twelve months, if not sooner. It can occur the day of release when the underlying biochemical cause has not been addressed and when the treatment facility has failed to provide healthy nutrition and nutritional education during the recovery process. Remember, hypoglycemia is a major reason for relapse.

When deciding which treatment program to go to, look for programs that provide the necessary elements that will lead to a relapse-free recovery.

Attempting addiction recovery without addressing imbalanced brain chemistry is like kayaking upstream without a paddle.

WHAT TO LOOK FOR

When choosing a facility for safe and rapid detoxification, with long term recovery goals, insist upon:

- IV therapy containing amino acids, vitamins, minerals and other nutrients
- Medications for detox symptoms, if needed, should be short term (3 to 5 days only)
- Education and focus on hypoglycemia
- Proper hydration (lots of water, no caffeine, sodas, etc.)
- Healthy nutrition and nutritional education including how to shop for food and supplements
- Education on how to manage an amino acid and co-factor protocol following discharge
- Daily exercise
- Daily infra-red saunas
- Massage
- Auricular therapy
- Acupuncture
- Yoga
- Meditation
- Music, dance, movement, art therapy
- Belief Management Training
- Integrative Memory Therapy®
- Support group
- No TV and computers, limited telephone use
- Minimum 90 days residency
- One year support and follow-up

At this time, only a few of these facilities exist in the U.S. but they must be the way of the future if we are to conquer this debilitating disorder.

♦ ♦ ♦

Thank you for reading this *Bottom Line Book*. Please share the information with others and help to save someone's life.   *Dr. Suka*

RESOURCES

SOME SUGGESTED LABORTORY TESTS

- CBC Complete Blood Count
- CMP Comprehensive Metabolic Panel
- A1c Test for diabetes and pre-diabetes
- Urinalysis
- Thyroid: TSH, Free T3, FreeT4
- 24 hour glucose tolerance test
- Hormone Levels
- Neurotransmitter levels
- Vitamin D level
- DHEA level
- Cortisol Level
- Copper/Zinc levels
- Toxic metals – Hair or blood analysis

SUGGESTED LABORTORIES

Direct Health: www.pyroluriatesting.com
Tests can be ordered directly by the individual on line, or through a healthcare provider. Insurance may cover these tests.

Sanesco Health: www.sanescohealth.com
Sanesco Health offers testing for neurotransmitters and adrenal insufficiency. (DHEA and Cortisol) Tests can be ordered through a healthcare provider. Insurance coverage is available.

NeuroScience: www.neurorelief.com
NeuroScience offers neurotransmitter testing. Tests can be ordered through a healthcare provider. Insurance coverage may be available.

Genova Diagnostics: www.gdx.net
Tests can be ordered through a healthcare provider. Insurance coverage may be available.

Life Extension: www.lef.org
Life Extension offers a large variety of tests available to the public without a prescription.

Vitamin D Council: www.vitamindcouncil.com
Inexpensive and accurate Vitamin D testing. No prescription necessary.

TO ORDER HIGH QUALITY SUPPLEMENTS LISTED IN THIS BOOK, CALL ANOVA HEALTH AT 864-408-8320.

Food supplements listed in all of our books can be purchased through Anova Health, also providing WHOLE FOOD supplements. Request a catalog.

Simply call Anova Health and give them the CODE. **Drsuka5** Your order will be shipped the same day, no delays. You will automatically receive a **5% discount and free shipping,** saving you the extra cost of buying supplements of the very best quality. To get these benefits, you must call in your order.

All supplements are of the highest quality available and are suitable for vegetarians. They are free of wheat gluten, soy, milk/dairy, corn, sodium, sugar, starch, artificial coloring, preservatives, and flavoring. I highly recommend the following supplements available through Anova Health.

Amino Acids: All of the amino acids that are listed in my two "how-to" manuals and other books can be ordered through Anova Health. Of course, they can be purchased in many other places, but for the highest quality and purest products, I recommend Anova Health. You may pay a little more, but you will use less and get better results with high quality products.

AvinoCort for managing elevated Cortisol levels caused by chronic stress. Lowering one's cortisol level slows down the aging process and helps to prevent dementia and Alzheimer's. Why use this product? This is a very advanced, stem cell product. Ask the folks at Anova Health for more information if you like. I highly recommend this product for reducing the effects of chronic stress.

Inositol Powder is a normal vitamin B. It is a precursor to GABA, the brain's natural Valium. If you have anxiety, worries, even panic attacks, your inositol level is probably too low. Taking 1000 mg up to four times daily can improve relaxation and reduce anxiety, naturally.

CaliQuil - California Poppy 500 mg Capsules Restores Rest. Prevails over pain. Traditional analgesic and sleep aid. This amazing product really works. Take it before bedtime and see the results. (Does not produce opium, physical dependence, or addiction.)

Acute Pain Relief, a King Bio homeopathic cream, gives excellent relief from joint pain.

Call 864-408-8320 to order these and other products from Anova Health. (If you order on-line, you won't get the discount or free shipping.)

Use the code **drsuka5** to order.

OTHER SUGGESTED RESOURCES FOR QUALITY SUPPLEMENTS
Call and request free catalogs. Order by telephone or on-line.

Life Extension: www.lef.org 1-800-678-8989

Bronson Vitamins: www.bronsonvitamins.com 1-800-235-3200

Cayenne Company: www.cayennecompany.com 1-800-229-3663

For highest quality amino acids call: Dr. Suka at 417-380-3254 or 417-894-8501

ARISE ALCOHOL RECOVERY, LLC PROGRAMS
Director: Suka Chapel-Horst, RN, PhD

Two Self-Help Recovery Programs that can take place in the comfort and privacy of one's home. These programs are based on biochemical restoration of the brain with micronutrient and nutrition therapy using the workbook *How to Quit Drinking for Good and Feel Good*.

- **Self-Managed Program** - Do it on your own following guidelines in the workbook.

- **Managed Program** which includes consultations with Dr. Suka.

Out-Patient Program: This program is based on biochemical restoration of the brain with micronutrient and nutrition therapy using the workbook *How to Quit Drinking for Good and Feel Good*. The out-patient program also includes approximately ten to fifteen sessions of *Integrative Memory Therapy*®.

For more information and testimonials, go to:
www.AriseAlcoholRecovery.com

RECOMMENDED BOOKS, DVDs

WORKBOOK   (180 pages)

How to Quit Drinking for Good and Feel Good

by Suka Chapel-Horst, RN, PhD, QMHP, CPLT

Live at Home

Keep it Private

Continue Normal Activities

Make it Affordable

Much of what we thought we knew about alcoholism and substance abuse is now obsolete. Neuroscience and biochemistry have found the underlying cause of all addictions and thirty-plus years of experience have given us the recovery method that is getting up to 85% recovery rates.

Shame, blame, and guilt be gone. Anger and hurt can change to healing, compassion and forgiveness when the real cause of addictions is understood. Addictions are not caused by a mental illness, nor are they caused by a lack of will power, a character defect, or a moral weakness.

Sobriety is not recovery. "One day at a time" struggling, white knuckling, dry drunk behaviors, depression, insomnia, anxiety, cravings, and other symptoms lead to relapse. With the new understanding of addictions, these, and other symptoms can be relieved and prevented, naturally, without the side effects and addictive qualities of prescription medications.

This book contains ten written tests to determine one's underlying biochemical imbalances, plus individual neurotransmitter tests, and a step-by-step guide for gaining and maintaining lasting recovery without the symptoms that lead to relapse. Normal brain chemistry is restored with the natural building blocks of amino acids, micronutrients and healthy nutrition. This program uses the most successful method of recovery available anywhere. Motivated and determined individuals can recover once and for all.

Written tests included in this book are:
- Alcohol Screening
- Carbohydrate Addiction
- Hypoglycemia
- Hypothyroid
- Candida
- Allergies
- Pyroluria
- High Histamine
- Low Histamine
- Attention Deficit (Hyperactivity) Disorder
- Neurotransmitter Deficiencies

DVD
Depression Cure
Ten Different Sources / Ten Different Approaches   Get Real Results
Your Guide to Finding and Treating the Real Underlying Cause
PowerPoint Presentation by Suka Chapel-Horst, RN, PhD, QMHP, CPLT

Don't waste time using the wrong approach to recovery. "Dr. Suka" pinpoints the different underlying sources of depression which must be treated uniquely and appropriately in order to fully recover without the use of pharmaceuticals. These inter-related causes require different treatment approaches to achieve permanent cure. Don't waste precious time, money, and hopes. Get to the root source from the start and find out how to recover naturally. DVD comes with a resource list.

WORKBOOK   (180 pages)
"Why Do I Feel This Way?" Natural Healing for Optimal Health and Relief from Moods and Depression
by Suka Chapel-Horst, RN, PhD, QMHP, CPLT

Moods, cravings, chronic depression, aches, pains and other symptoms are caused by treatable and reversible deficiencies in brain chemistry.

If your brain is low in "feel good" chemicals, you may experience moodiness, sadness, anxiety, overeating, insomnia, irritability, anger, lack of focus and concentration, poor memory, loneliness, decreased sex drive, lack of motivation, racing thoughts, suicidal thoughts, and more.

Find out which "feel good" brain chemicals you may be deficient in. Experience the power of amino acids to restore brain chemistry without medications. Discover the foods and basic food supplements that can restore your life to normal. The guidelines are clear, easy to understand and follow. This book may be all you need to achieve optimal health.

Avoid medication side effects, serious dangers, and addictive qualities. The only way to restore optimal health is by deleting poisonous nonfoods and feeding the brain the natural substances it needs to function normally.

The book includes:
- Ten Written Tests to Uncover the Underlying Cause
- Neurotransmitter Testing
- Amino Acid Formulas
- Nutritional Co-Factor Formulas
- Three Nutritional Programs
- Allergy and Candida Repair
- Seventeen Fun and Effective Stress-Reducing Exercises

BOOK (234 pages)
Take a Leap of Faith
Wellness Simplified
by Suka Chapel-Horst, RN, PhD, QMHP, CPLT

If your emotional, mental, or physical health isn't what you wish it to be, you'll find practical suggestions for regaining or maintaining optimal health in this remarkable book. The topics include:

- Halt Premature Aging Now
- Want More Sunshine in Your Life?
- The Cookie Monster - Hypoglycemia
- Five Simple Steps to Optimal Health
- Enjoy Life More
- Your Body Type: Seven Dwarfs and Superman
- Fear versus Love
- Relief from Depression
- Stretching to Wellness
- Bodyguards Got You Covered?
- Bodyguard Banquet
- What are you Hoarding in your Mental House?
- Prevent Dementia and Alzheimer's
- The Hundredth Monkey Cure – Cannabinoids
- Is There a Cure for Alcoholism?
- Color – The Hidden Persuader
- The Ultimate Healing – Integrative Memory Therapy®
- Take a Leap of Faith
- What I know for Sure
- ...and more

In the most delightful and warm way, Dr. Suka "talks" about the topics closest to our minds and hearts. This book includes transcripts from 24 of her recent Unity.FM international radio shows. You won't want to put this book down.

BOTTOM LINE BOOKS

BOOK/DVD
Wellness Simplified
How Food affects Moods, Bodies and Behaviors
PowerPoint Presentation by Suka Chapel-Horst, RN, PhD, QMHP, CPLT

Think what you eat doesn't matter? Fast food, junk food, sodas, and pizza are the voices of violence, crime, and suicide, as well as obesity, joint pain, insomnia, anxiety, diabetes, depression, cancer, and *you name it!*

What we eat affects the quality of our lives. Sick and tired of feeling sick and tired? Are children's behaviors getting out of hand? Are school grades going down? It's OK. There's a solution and it's not rocket science.

This little book can change lives for the better, right now. The solution makes sense and it's doable. Say "goodbye" to moods, sickness, and unwanted behaviors. Say "hello" to good health and happiness.

BOOK/DVD
Say Goodbye to Moods and Depression
PowerPoint Presentation by Suka Chapel-Horst, RN, PhD, QMHP, CPLT

The only way to restore optimal health is by deleting poisonous nonfoods and feeding the brain the natural substances from which it is made.

Babies are made from food, not Prozac. After birth, why do we switch from the natural building blocks of life to synthetic pills? We can achieve optimal health when we remove the underlying brain chemical imbalances which lead to the symptoms of moods and depression including insomnia, anxiety, panic reactions, irritability, weight gain, aches and pains, and more.

The good news is that targeted micronutrients and healthy nutrition, along with other holistic methods of healthcare, can reduce or eliminate moods and depression, naturally.

BOOK/DVD
PTSD – Post-Traumatic Stress Disorder
Alternative Resources for Recovery
PowerPoint Presentation by Suka Chapel-Horst, RN, PhD, QMHP, CPLT

Medications have long term, harmful side effects, including addiction, and traditional counseling methods are often only partially effective.

There are two underlying causes of PTSD. 1) Biochemical deficiencies, or brain chemistry imbalances, and 2) underlying, UNCONSCIOUS, unresolved trauma which occurred PRIOR to the known trauma-experience that *appears* to be the cause of PTSD. These unconscious memories are called *source trauma.*

Addressing biochemical, nutritional, brain wave state, and bioenergy fields is a necessary component to recovery, including the clearing of destructive cellular memories using the latest science of energy psychology.

Uncovering and resolving hidden source trauma, the underlying cause of PTSD, is accomplished with *Integrative Memory Therapy®.*

BOOK/DVD
The Gift – A Sound Mind for Life
PowerPoint Presentation by Suka Chapel-Horst, RN, PhD, QMHP, CPLT

How to increase mental focus, improve memory, and prevent or delay Alzheimer's. Find out about the effects of stress and how to minimize it in order to prolong health and quality life. The DVD includes biochemical, nutritional, physical, emotional, and mental resources to minimize and delay the effects of aging. This is valuable information for any age.

BOOK/DVD

Cannabinoids – The Hundredth Monkey Cure

A PowerPoint Presentation by Suka Chapel-Horst, RN, PhD, QMHP, CPLT

The human body naturally produces cannabis-like chemicals that keep all body systems in balance. This internal cannabinoid system may be the most important health discovery of recent years. THC, CBN, and CBD from the cannabis sativa plant mimic our internal chemicals and work to improve our overall health. Cannabidiol, or CBD, cures or relieves symptoms of over 100 disorders. ...and it's legal everywhere because it doesn't have the psycho-active ingredient, THC.

Want better natural solutions for your health concerns? This DVD shows how to change brain chemistry and improve your life by using Cannabidiol (CBD), amino acids, neuro-nutrients, nutrition, exercise, and chronic stress reducers. Say goodbye to anxiety, stress, depression, insomnia, pain, physical disorders, and much more.

BOOK/DVD

Trick or Treat – What Your Doctor isn't Telling You about Mood Altering Medications

PowerPoint Presentation by Suka Chapel-Horst, RN, PhD, QMHP, CPLT

Is your doctor treating you or tricking you? If you are considering taking mood altering medications, are already on them, or want to get off them, you need to know what these medications are really doing to brain chemistry. Be informed in order to make wise decisions. Your emotional and mental life is at stake.

BOOK/DVD

These books and DVDs can be ordered through:
www.AriseAlcoholRecovery.com
www.IMRIWellness.org
Or by calling: 417-380-3254

Suka Chapel-Horst

www.ingramcontent.com/pod-product-compliance
Lightning Source LLC
Chambersburg PA
CBHW070322290526
45791CB00003B/1217